Say It Rite: Quick Reference Guide of Controlled Substances CII-CV

Author
Zachery P. Post CPhT.

References: Globalrph.com
Mims.com
Wikipedia.org
Drugs.com
The Pill Book – 12th Ed.
Facts and Comparisons
MedicineNet.com

Published By
Say It Rite

ISBN-13: 978-0-9820215-1-4

Printed in the U.S.A
WWW.SAYITRITE.COM

This guide has been created for every nurse, cna, p.a., pharmacy technician, and anyone studying or working in the medical field. It is the must have guide packed with over 100+ controlled substances picked from the DEA list of controlled substances. Also it has a list of the top 200 medications used in the U.S., and a conversion/ measurement table, and the break down of many medical abbreviations. This is the guide for you, if you want to distinguish between controlled and non-controlled medications, learn why certain medication or placed at certain levels of control, and spend less time looking for medications around your pharmacy.

Note: This guide is intended to help educate and not to be used as a substitute for a physician's knowledge. Only a physician can give prescriptions for these medications and their exact dosage. Some medications on this list have been pulled off the market, but are still found on the DEA controlled substance list.

Table of Contents:

Controlled Substance Schedule

The Controlled Substances Act of 1970, as amended, places certain restrictions on substances that have potential for abuse. These substances have been placed in categories according to their potential for abuse.

(1) Schedule I. –

(A) The drug or other substance has a high potential for abuse.
(B) The drug or other substance has no currently accepted medical use in treatment in the United States.
(C) There is a lack of accepted safety for use of the drug or other substance under medical supervision.
(2) Schedule II. –

(A) The drug or other substance has a high potential for abuse.
(B) The drug or other substance has a currently accepted medical use in treatment in the United

States or a currently accepted medical use with severe restrictions.

(C) Abuse of the drug or other substances may lead to severe psychological or physical dependence.

(3) Schedule III. –

(A) The drug or other substance has a potential for abuse less than the drugs or other substances in schedules I and II.(B) The drug or other substance has a currently accepted medical use in treatment in the United States.

(C) Abuse of the drug or other substance may lead to moderate or low physical dependence or high psychologicaldependence.

(4) Schedule IV. –

(A) The drug or other substance has a low potential for abuse relative to the drugs or other substances in schedule III.

(B) The drug or other substance has a currently accepted medical use in treatment in the United States.

(C) Abuse of the drug or other substance may lead to limited physical dependence or psychological dependence relative to the drugs or other substances in schedule III.
(5) Schedule V. –

(A) The drug or other substance has a low potential for abuse relative to the drugs or other substances in schedule IV.
(B) The drug or other substance has a currently accepted medical use in treatment in the United States.
(C) Abuse of the drug or other substance may lead to limited physical dependence or psychological dependence relative to the drugs or other substances in schedule IV.

4

**ALFENTANIL
HYDROCHLORIDE –CII
(ALFENTA)**
Prescribed For: The maintenance of anesthesia with barbiturate/nitrous oxide/oxygen.
**Drug Class: OPIOID
ANALGESIC**
Usual Dosage: For the induction of analgesia in adults: 8-20 mcg/kg, and for the maintenance of analgesia in adults the dosage is 3-5 mcg/kg every 5-20 min or 0.5 to 1 mcg/kg/min.
Side Effects: Include respiratory depression and skeletal muscle rigidity.

**ALPHAPRODINE-CII (Nisentil
and Prisilidine)**
Prescribed For: Pain relief in childbirth, dentistry, and as well as for minor surgical procedures.

5

Drug Class: OPIOID ANALGESIC

Usual Dosage: Should be individualized and titrated to the desired effect in each patient according to body weight and physical status.

Side Effects: Include itching, nausea and potentially serious respiratory depression which can be life-threatening.

AMOBARBITAL-CII (AMYLOBARBITONE)

Prescribed For: sedative-hypnotic

Drug Class: BARBITURATE DERIVATIVE

Usual Dosage: For adults with sleeping trouble the dosage is 65mg-200mg at bedtime, for daytime sedation it is 50mg-300mg smaller doses taken in the day. For sedation before surgery 200mg one to two hours before surgery.

Side Effects: Include confusion (severe), decrease in or loss of reflexes, drowsiness (severe), fever, irritability (continuing), low body temperature, poor judgment, shortness of breath or slow or troubled breathing, and slow heartbeat.

COCAINE HYDROCHLORIDE-CII (COCAINE)

Prescribed For: The introduction of local (topical) anesthesia of accessible mucous membranes of the oral, laryngeal and nasal cavities.

Drug Class: Crystalline Tropane Alkaloid

Usual Dosage: The usual adult dosage varies and depends upon the area to be anesthetized, vascularity of the tissues, individual tolerance, and the technique of anesthesia.

Side Effects: The most common side effects are dizziness, nausea, nervousness, unusual feelings of well-being, and restlessness.

CODEINE-CII (CODEINE)

Prescribed For: The relief of mild to moderate pain.

Drug Class: Opioid Analgesic

Usual Dosage: The usual adult dosage is 15mg-60mg orally every 4 hours as needed.

Side Effects: The most common side effects are lightheadedness, dizziness, sedation, nausea, vomiting, and sweating, and respiratory depression.

DEXTROPROPOXYPHENE-CII
Prescribed For: The relief of mild to moderate pain.
Drug Class: Opioid Analgesic
Usual Dosage: The usual adult dosage is 100mg orally four times a day as needed.
Side Effects: The most common side effects are stomach pains, nausea, and vomiting, dry mouth, decreased appetite, urinary retention and constipation.

DIHYDROCODEINE-CII (DHC, Drocode, Paracodeine and Parzone)
Prescribed For: The treatment of postoperative pain, severe dyspnea, or as an antitussive.
Drug Class: Opioid Analgesic

Usual Dosage: The usual adult dosage is 16mg-32mg orally every 4-6 hours as needed.
Side Effects: Tolerance and physical and psychological dependence develop with repeated. Others include giddiness, sense of hyperactivity, itching, flushing, and constipation.

DIHYDROETORPHINE-CII
Prescribed For: The relief of moderate to severe pain.
Drug Class: Semi-Synthetic Opioid
Usual Dosage: The usual adult doses range from 20mg to 180mg orally or intravenously.
Side Effects: The most common side effects are dizziness, sedation, nausea, constipation, and respiratory depression.

DIPRENORPHINE-CII
(Revivon, M5050)
Prescribed For: To reverse the effects of super-potent opioid analgesics. (Ex. etorphine and carfentanil)
Drug Class: Opioid Antagonist

Usual Dosage: Dosage varies depending on the height, weight, and other physical characteristics.
Side Effects: The most common side effect is respiratory depression.

ETHYLMORPHINE-CII (Codethyline, Dionine)
Prescribed For: An antitussive for the treatment of dry cough, and also ophthalmology for removing inflammation products from the eyes, and also inducing miosis.
Drug Class: Opioid Analgesic
Usual Dosage: Dosages range from 5mg to 50mg intravenously.
Side Effects: The most common side effects are nausea, vomiting, urinary retention, miosis, constipation, and psychological addiction.

ETORPHINE-CII (Immobilon or M99)
Prescribed For: The immobilization of large mammals.
Drug Class: Semi-Synthetic Opioid

Usual Dosage: Dosage varies depending on the height, weight, and other physical characteristics.
Side Effects: The most common side effects are mild hyperventilation, cardiac arrhythmias, endocarditis, or hepatic impairment.

**FENTANYL-CII
(DURAGESIC®)**
Prescribed For: The control of persistent moderate to severe chronic pain that needs around the clock treatment.
Drug Class: Opioid Agonist
Usual Dosage: The usual dosage ranges from 25mcg patch to 300mcg patches applied topical every 72 hours. Patients using fentanyl should be opioid-tolerant and receiving at least 60 mg of oral morphine equivalents per day.
Side Effects: The most common side effects are abdominal pain, headache, fatigue, back pain, fever, influenza-like symptoms, accidental injury, rigors, nausea, vomiting, dry mouth, constipation, insomnia and euphoria.

GLUTETHIMIDE-CII (Doriden)
Prescribed For: The treatment of insomnia.
Drug Class: Hypnotic Sedative
Usual Dosage: The usual adult dosage is 500mg orally at bedtime. Doses may vary depending on the patient's condition.
Side Effects: The most common side effects are blurred vision, clumsiness or unsteadiness, confusion, dizziness, headache, nausea, vomiting, and also daytime drowsiness.

HYDROCODONE-CII (Hycodan)
Prescribed For: The relief of pain and also as a cough suppressant.
Drug Class: Semi-Synthetic Opioid Derived
Usual Dosage: The usual adult dose ranges from 5mg-10mg orally.
Side Effects: The most common side effects are dizziness, lightheadedness, nausea, drowsiness, constipation, vomiting, and euphoria.

HYDROMORPHONE HYDROCHLORIDE –CII (DILAUDID®)

Prescribed For: The management of pain.

Drug Class: Opioid Analgesic

Usual Dosage: The usual adult dosage is 2mg-4mg orally every 4-6 hours. For the oral liquid it is 2.5ml-10ml every 3-6 hours.

Side Effects: The most common side effects are light-headedness, dizziness, sedation, nausea, vomiting, sweating, flushing, dysphoria, euphoria, dry mouth, and pruritus.

LEVORPHANOL-CII (Levo-Dromoran)

Prescribed For: For the treatment of severe pain.

Drug Class: Opioid Agonists

Usual Dosage: The usual adult dosage is 2mg-4mg orally or subcutaneous injection every 6-8 hours.

Side Effects: The most common side effects are nausea, vomiting, constipation, loss of appetite, dizziness, headache, tired feeling, dry mouth, loss of interest in sex, sweating, and itching.

MEPERIDINE-CII (Demerol®)
Prescribed For: The relief of moderate to severe pain.
Drug Class: Opioid Analgesic
Usual Dosage: The usual dosage is 50mg- 150mg orally every 3-4 hours as needed.
Side Effects: The most common side effects are lightheadedness, dizziness, sedation, nausea, vomiting, and sweating.

METHADONE-CII (DOLOPHINE®)
Prescribed For: The treatment of moderate to severe pain when no reaction to non- narcotic analgesics. Also for detoxification treatment of opioid addiction (heroin or other morphine-like drugs).
Drug Class: Opioid Agonists
Usual Dosage: The usual adult dosage is 2.5 mg to 10 mg every 8 to 12 hours, and slowly increase or decrease due to effect.
Side Effects: The most common side effects are lightheadedness,

dizziness, sedation, nausea, vomiting, and sweating, headaches, weakness, and edema.

METHYLPHENIDATE HYDROCHLORIDE -CII (CONCERTA, RITALIN, METHYLIN)

Prescribed For: The treatment of attention deficit disorders, and narcolepsy.

Drug Class: Mild Central Nervous System Stimulant (CNS)

Usual Dosage: The usual adult dosage is 20mg-30mg orally in divided doses 2-3 times a day. The usual dosage for children is 5mg orally twice a day and may increase by 5mg-10mg weekly.

Side Effects: The most common side effects are nervousness, insomnia, anorexia, nausea, dizziness, palpitations, headache, dyskinesia, and drowsiness.

MORPHINE-CII (AVINZA®)

Prescribed For: The relief of moderate to severe pain that needs around the clock treatment.

Drug Class: Opioid Agonists

15

Usual Dosage: The usual adult dosage is 30mg orally once a day and increased due to effect.
Side Effects: The most common side effects are vomiting, nausea, dehydration, dyspnea, and sepsis.

NABILONE-CII (CESAMET™)
Prescribed for: The treatment of nausea and vomiting for patients receiving cancer chemotherapy.
Drug Class: Synthetic Cannabinoid
Usual Dosage: The usual adult dose is 1mg-2mg orally twice a day. On the days of chemotherapy it should be given 1-3 hours before treatment begins.
Side Effects: The most common side effects are drowsiness, vertigo, dry mouth, euphoria, ataxia, headache, and concentration difficulties.

OPIUM TINCTURE-CII (Laudanum)
Prescribed For: Treatment of diarrhea, and pain relief.
Drug Class: Analgesic and Antidiarrheal

Usual Dosage: The usual adult dosage is 0.3-1 mL orally every 2-6 hours to maximum of 6 mL orally with in 24 hours. The usual dosage for children is 0.005-0.01 mL/kg orally every 3-4 hours for a maximum of 6 doses orally with in 24 hours

Side Effects: The most common side effects are dizziness and drowsiness, restlessness, insomnia or depression.

OXYCODONE HYDROCHLORIDE-CII (ROXICODONE®)

Prescribed For: The relief of moderate to severe pain.

Drug Class: Opioid Analgesic

Usual Dosage: The usual adult dosage is 10mg-30mg orally every 4 hours as needed for pain.

Side Effects: The most common side effects are constipation, dizziness, drowsiness, headache, nausea, sleeplessness, vomiting, and weakness.

OXYCODONE WITH ACETAMINOPHEN-CII (Endocet, Percocet)

17

Prescribed For: The relief of moderate to moderately severe pain.

Drug Class: Opioid Analgesic

Usual Dosage: The usual adult dosage is 1 tablet orally every 6 hours as needed for pain the total daily dose of acetaminophen should not be over 4grams.

Side Effects: The most common side effects are lightheadedness, dizziness, drowsiness or sedation, nausea, and vomiting.

PENTOBARBITAL-CII (NEMBUTAL®)

Prescribed For: The use as a sedative, preanesthetic, for short-term treatment of insomnia, and as an anticonvulsant.

Drug Class: Barbiturates

Usual Dosage: The usual dosage varies due to height, weight, and physical condition, but the most commonly used starting dose for an adult that is 70kg is 100mg.

Side Effects: The most common side effects are agitation, confusion, hyperkinesia, ataxia, CNS depression, nightmares, nervousness, psychiatric disturbance, hallucinations, insomnia, anxiety, dizziness, and thinking abnormality.

PHENCYCLIDINE-CII (PCP)
Prescribed For: An anesthetic in surgery.
Drug Class: Anesthetic Agent
Usual Dosage: This medication was pulled from the market in 1963, but is used as a street drug for recreational use.
Side Effects: The most common side effects are hallucinations, mania, delirium, and disorientation.

PHENMETRAZINE TARTRATE-CII (BONTRIL®)
Prescribed For: The management of exogenous obesity.
Drug Class: Weight control supplement
Usual Dosage: The usual adult dosage is 35mg orally twice a day or three times a day one hour before meals.
Side Effects: The most common side effects are over stimulation, restlessness, insomnia, agitation, flushing, tremor, sweating, dizziness, headache, psychotic state, blurring of vision, diarrhea,

nausea, constipation, and stomach ache.

REMIFENTANIL HYDROCHLORIDE -CII (ULTIVA®)
Prescribed for: An analgesic agent for use during the induction and maintenance of general anesthesia for inpatient and outpatient procedures.
Drug Class: Opioid Analgesic
Usual Dosage: The usual dosage varies due to height, weight, and physical condition, but the usual adult dosage is based on 0.5 to 1 mcg/kg/min.
Side Effects: The most common side effects are respiratory depression, bradycardia, hypotension, and skeletal muscle rigidity.

SECOBARBITAL-CII (Seconal)
Prescribed For: A short acting sedative.
Drug Class: Barbiturate Derivative

Usual Dosage: The usual adult dosage range in concentrations from 8mg-250mg.

Side Effects: The most common side effects are somnolence, dizziness, anxiety, confusion, headache, nausea, vomiting, nightmares, anxiety, and insomnia.

SUFENTANIL CITRATE -CII (SUFENTA®)

Prescribed For: An analgesic adjunct in the maintenance of balanced general anesthesia.

Drug Class: Opioid Analgesic

Usual Dosage: The usual dosage varies due to height, weight, and physical condition.

Side Effect: The most common side effects are respiratory depression and skeletal muscle rigidity.

ACETAMINOPHEN WITH CODEINE-CIII (Tylenol with Codeine)

Prescribed For: The relief of mild to moderately severe pain.

Drug Class: Opioid Analgesic

Usual Dosage: The usual adult dosage is 15mg-60mg of codeine

and 300mg-1000mg of acetaminophen orally every 4 hours.
Side Effects: The most common side effects are euphoria, constipation, drowsiness, lightheadedness, dizziness, sedation, shortness of breath, nausea and vomiting.

BENZPHETAMINE-CIII (Didrex)
Prescribed For: The short-term management of exogenous obesity.
Drug Class: Weight Loss Supplement
Usual Dosage: The usual adult dosage should start with 25mg-50mg orally one to three times a day. Then increased according to patient's response.
Side Effects: The most common side effects are over stimulation, restlessness, dizziness, insomnia, tremor, sweating, and headache.

BUTABARBITAL-CIII (BUTISOL SODIUM®)
Prescribed For: Short-term treatment of insomnia.

22

Drug Class: CSN Depressant
Usual Dosage: The usual adult dosage for daytime sedative is 15mg-30mg orally 3-4 times a day, as for a bedtime hypnotic it is 50mg-100mg at bedtime, and for preoperative sedative - 50 to 100 mg 60-90 minutes before surgery.
Side Effects: The most common side effects are somnolence, headache, and dependence.

BUTOBARBITAL-CIII
(Soneryl®)
Prescribed For: Treatment of severe insomnia.
Drug Class: Barbiturate
Usual Dosage: The usual adult dosage is 1-2 100mg tablets orally at bedtime.
Side Effects: The most common side effects are drowsiness, headache, unsteadiness, and incoordination.

DRONABINOL-CIII
(MARINOL®)
Prescribed For: The control of weight loss in patients with HIV or for the relief of nausea and

vomiting in patients receiving chemotherapy.

Drug Class: Appetite Stimulate and also a Mild Opioid Analgesic

Usual Dosage: The usual adult dosage is 2.5mg orally twice a day before lunch and dinner.

Side Effects: The most common side effects are asthenia, anxiety/nervousness, thinking abnormal, dizziness, euphoria, and abdominal pain.

DROSTANOLONE PROPIONATE -CIII (Masteron)

Prescribed For: The treatment of breast cancer.

Drug Class: Anabolic Steroid

Usual Dosage: The usual adult dosage is 167mgs/kg-bdywt/day.

Side Effects: The most common side effects are acne, accelerated hair loss, and increased aggression.

EMBUTRAMIDE-CIII (Embutane)

Prescribed For: A sedative before surgery.

Drug Class: General Anesthetic Agent

Usual Dosage: The usual adult dosage is 50mg/kg intravenously. It is mainly used in euthanizing dogs.

Side Effects: The most common side effects are respiratory depression and ventricular arrhythmia.

FLUOXYMESTERONE-CII (Halotestin)
Prescribed For: The treatment of male hypogonadism, delayed puberty in males, and in the treatment of breast neoplasms in women.

Drug Class: Anabolic Steroid
Usual Dosage: The usual adult dosage for men is 5mg-20mg orally daily, and for women it is 10mg-40mg orally daily.

Side Effects: The most common side effects in women are amenorrhea and other menstrual irregularities; inhibition of gonadotropin secretion; and virilization, including deepening of the voice and clitoral enlargement. In men gynecomastia and excessive frequency and duration of penile erections.

25

FORMEBOLONE-CIII
(Esiclene)
Prescribed For: The treatment of children deficient in growth.

Drug Class: Anabolic Steroid
Usual Dosage: The usual dosage varies depending on physical conditions of patient and should be determined by a physician.
Side Effects: The most common side effects are usually pain at the injection site.

FURAZABOL-CIII (Miotolan)
Prescribed For: The long-term treatment of arteriosclerosis and hypercholesterolemia.
Drug Class: Anabolic Steroid Derivative
Usual Dosage: The usual recommended daily dose is 2-6 mg.
Side Effects: The most common side effects include an increase in aggression, acne and an unwanted body hair.

HYDROCODONE BITARTRATE WITH ACETAMINOPHEN-CIII

(Lortab, Vicoden, Lorcet and Norco)
Prescribed For: The relief of moderate to moderately severe pain.
Drug Class: Semi-Synthetic Opioid Analgesic
Usual Dosage: The usual adult dosage is 1-2 tablets orally every 4-6 hours as needed for pain.
Side Effects: The most common side effects are constipation light-headedness, dizziness, sedation, nausea and vomiting.

KETAMINE HYDROCHLORIDE –CIII
Prescribed For: The sole anesthetic agent for diagnostic and surgical procedures that do not require skeletal muscle relaxation.
Drug Class: Anesthetic Agent
Usual Dosage: The usual adult dosage is 2mg/kg intravenous before surgery.
Side Effects: The most common side effects are severe depression of respiration or apnea, hypotension, bradycardia, nausea and vomiting.

METHENOLONE ACETATE-CIII (Primobolan)

Prescribed For: Aid in the reducing breast tumors.

Drug Class: Anabolic Steroid

Usual Dosage: The usual adult male dosage is 200mg-300mg orally a day, and women should not exceed 30mg orally a day.

Side Effects: The most common side effect is hair loss.

METHYPRYLON-CIII

Prescribed For: The treatment of insomnia.

Drug Class: Piperidinedione Derivative

Usual Dosage: The usual adult dosage is 300mg orally at bedtime.

Side Effects: The most common side effects are confusion, rapid heartbeat, drowsiness, shortness of breath, swelling of feet and lower legs, and weakness.

OXANDROLONE-CIII (Oxandrin)

Prescribed For: The treatment of alcoholic hepatitis, Turner's syndrome, and weight loss caused by HIV.

Drug Class: Anabolic Steroid
Usual Dosage: The usual adult dosage is 2.5mg-20mg orally given in 2-4 divided doses daily.
Side Effects: The most common side effects in males are phallic enlargement and increased frequency or persistence of erections, also inhibition of testicular function, testicular atrophy and oligospermia, impotence, chronic priapism, epididymitis, and bladder irritability. In females clitoral enlargement, and menstrual irregularities.

OXYMETHOLONE-CIII (ANADROL®)
Prescribed For: The treatment of anemia's caused by deficient red cell production.
Drug Class: Anabolic Steroid
Usual Dosage: The usual adult dosage is 1-5mg per kg body weight daily.
Side Effects: The most common side effects in males are phallic enlargement and increased

frequency or persistence of erections, and in female's clitoral enlargement, and menstrual irregularities. In insomnia, nausea, vomiting, and diarrhea.

STANOZOLOL-CIII (WINSTROL)
Prescribed For: Prophylactically to decrease the frequency and severity of attacks of angioedema.
Drug Class: Anabolic Steroid
Usual Dosage: The usual adult doses is to start at 2mg orally three times a day then should be decreased due to reaction of patients condition.
Side Effects: The most common side effects are habituation, excitation, insomnia, and depression in both sexes and in female's clitoral enlargement, and menstrual irregularities. In male's phallic enlargement and increased frequency of erections.

TESTOLACTONE-CIII (TESLAC®)
Prescribed For: Adjunctive therapy in the palliative treatment

of advanced or disseminated breast cancer in postmenopausal women when hormonal therapy is needed.

Drug Class: Anabolic Steroid
Usual Dosage: The usual adult dosage is 250mg orally four times a day.

Side Effects: The most common side effects are maculopapular erythema, increase in blood pressure, paresthesia, malaise, aches and edema of the extremities, glossitis, anorexia, nausea and vomiting.

TESTOSTERONE GEL 1%-CIII (AndroGel®)

Prescribed For: Replacement therapy in adult males for conditions associated with a deficiency or absence of endogenous testosterone.

Drug Class: Androgen
Usual Dosage: The usual adult dosage is to start as 5gm once a day topically to the shoulders and upper arms or abdomen.

Side Effects: The most common side effects are acne, depression, prostate disorder, drowsiness, nervousness, and alopecia.

THIOPENTAL-CIII (Pentothal)
Prescribed For: The sole anesthetic agent for brief (15 minute) procedures.
Drug Class: Thiobarbiturate
Usual Dosage: The adult test dosage is 25mg-75mg intravenous, and should be dosed according to the patient's weight and reaction to test dose by physician.
Side Effects: The most common side effects are respiratory depression, myocardial depression, cardiac arrhythmias, prolonged somnolence and recovery, sneezing, coughing, bronchospasm, laryngospasm and shivering.

ALPRAZOLAM-CIV (XANAX®)
Prescribed For: The management of anxiety disorder, or the short-term relief of symptoms of anxiety.
Drug Class: Benzodiazepine
Usual Dosage: The usual adult dosage is 0.25mg to 0.5mg given orally three times daily with the

maximum daily dose of 4 mg, given in divided doses.

Side Effects: The most common side effects are drowsiness or light-headedness, depression, headache, confusion, insomnia, constipation, diarrhea, nausea and vomiting.

BROMAZEPAM-CIV (Lexotan, Brazepam, and Bromaze)
Prescribed For: The management of anxiety disorder.
Drug Class: Benzodiazepine Derivative
Usual Dosage: The usual adult dosage is 6mg-18mg orally in a day given in divided doses.
Side Effects: The most common side effects are drowsiness, sedation, muscle weakness and ataxia; less frequently vertigo, headache, confusion, depression, slurred speech, changes in libido, tremor, visual disturbances, and urinary retention.

BUTORPHANOL-CIV (STADOL ®)
Prescribed For: A preoperative or preanesthetic medication, as a supplement to balanced anesthesia,

33

and for the relief of pain during labor.

Drug Class: Synthetically Derived Opioid Agonist-Antagonist Analgesic

Usual Dosage: The usual adult single dose for intravenous administration is 1 mg repeated every 3 to 4 hours as necessary. The effective dosage range, depending on the severity of pain, is 0.5 to 2 mg repeated every 3 to 4 hours.

Side Effects: The most common side effects are sedation, dizziness, physical dependence, with or without psychological dependence; dyspnoea, confusion, headache, nausea, vomiting, drowsiness, constipation; hallucinations, mental depression, HTN and paradoxical CNS excitation (especially in children); rash, syncope, tinnitus, vertigo, and diaphoresis.

CHLORAL BETAINE-CIV (Welldorm)
Prescribed For: Short-term treatment of insomnia.
Drug Class: Sedatives

Usual Dosage: The usual adult dose is 1-2 tablets orally 15-30 minutes before bedtime.

Side Effects: The most common side effects are gastric irritation, abdominal distension and flatulence, allergic skin reactions, headache and ketonuria.

CHLORDIAZEPOXIDE-CIV (LIBRIUM®)

Prescribed For: The management of anxiety disorders or for the short term relief of symptoms of anxiety, withdrawal" symptoms of acute alcoholism, and preoperative apprehension and anxiety.

Drug Class:
Psychopharmacologic Compound

Usual Dosage: The usual adult dose is 5mg-25mg orally two to four times a day.

Side Effects: The most common side effects are drowsiness, ataxia, confusion and syncope.

CLOBAZAM –CIV (Frisium)

Prescribed For: Tonic-clonic, complex partial, myoclonic seizures, and certain types of status epilepticus.

Drug Class: Long acting Benzodiazepine
Usual Dosage: The usual adult dosage is 20-30 mg orally daily in divided doses or as a single dose given at night.
Side Effects: The most common side effects are drowsiness, dizziness, tiredness, fatigue, loss of coordination, nausea, constipation, loss of appetite, muscle weakness, dry mouth, tremor, weight gain, or restlessness.

CLONAZEPAM-CIV (Klonopin)
Prescribed For: The treatment of panic disorder and Lennox-Gastaut syndrome.
Drug Class: Benzodiazepine
Usual Dosage: The usual adult's dosage for seizure disorder is 1.5 mg/day orally divided into three doses and should not be exceeded. For panic disorder the dosage is 0.25mg orally two times a day.
Side Effects: The most common side effects are abnormal eye movements, depression, headache, tremor, vertigo, dizziness, nervousness, somnolence and ataxia.

CLORAZEPATE DIPOTASSIUM –CIV (TRANXENE* T-TAB®)

Prescribed For: The treatment of anxiety, acute alcohol withdrawal, and seizures.

Drug Class: Benzodiazepine

Usual Dosage: The usual adult dosage is 30mg orally daily given in divided doses.

Side Effects: The most common side effects are drowsiness, dizziness, fatigue, dry mouth, upset stomach, constipation, blurred vision, or headache.

DEXFENFLURAMINE HYDROCHLORIDE –CIV (Redux)

Prescribed For: The management of obesity including weight loss and maintenance of weight loss in patients on a reduced calorie diet.

Drug Class: Serotonin Reuptake Inhibitor

Usual Dosage: The usual adult dosage is 15mg capsule orally twice a day with meals.

Side Effects: The most common side effects are diarrhea, dry mouth, and somnolence.

DIAZEPAM-CIV (VALIUM)
Prescribed For: The management of anxiety disorders or for the short-term relief of the symptoms of anxiety.
Drug Class: Benzodiazepine Derivative
Usual Dosage: For the management of anxiety the usual adult dosage is 2mg-10mg orally two to four times daily in divided doses.
Side Effects: The most common side effects are drowsiness, fatigue, muscle weakness, ataxia, depression, headaches, tremors, restlessness, constipation, nausea, and dizziness.

DIETHYLPROPION-CIV (TENUATE®)
Prescribed For: The short-term management of exogenous obesity.
Drug Class: Weight loss-supplement

Usual Dosage: The usual adult dosage is one immediate-release 25 mg tablet three times daily, one hour before meals and in mid-evening if desired to overcome night hunger.

Side Effects: The most common side effects are elevation of blood pressure, blurred vision, over stimulation, nervousness, restlessness, dizziness, jitteriness, insomnia, anxiety, euphoria, depression, dysphoria, vomiting, diarrhea, abdominal discomfort, and dry mouth.

DIFENOXIN WITH ATROPINE SULFATE-CIV (Motofen)
Prescribed For: Adjunctive therapy in the management of acute nonspecific diarrhea and acute exacerbations of chronic functional diarrhea.

Drug Class: Antidiarrheal Agent
Usual Dosage: The most usual adult starting dosage is 2mg orally then 1mg orally every loose stool and every 3-4 hours as needed.

Side Effects: The most common side effects are nausea, vomiting, dizziness, constipation, dry mouth, lightheadedness, and drowsiness.

ESTAZOLAM-CIV (Prosom)
Prescribed For: The short-term management of insomnia characterized by difficulty in falling asleep, frequent nocturnal awakenings, and/or early morning awakenings.
Drug Class: Triazolobenzodiazepine Derivative
Usual Dosage: The usual adult dosage is 1mg orally at bedtime.
Side Effects: The most common side effects are clumsiness or unsteadiness, daytime drowsiness, dizziness, fatigue, feeling of hangover, headache, lightheadedness, nausea, nervousness, sluggishness, and unusual weakness.

ETHCHLORVYNOL-CIV (Placidyl)
Prescribed For: The short-term treatment of insomnia.
Drug Class: Sedative-Hypnotic Tertiary Carbinols

Usual Dosage: The usual adult dosage is 500mg-1000mg orally at bedtime.

Side Effects: The most common side effects are skin rash, restlessness, drowsiness, faintness, and unusual excitement.

ETHINAMATE-CIV (Valamin, Valmid)
Prescribed For: The short-term treatment of insomnia.
Drug Class: Benzodiazepine Hypnotic Agent
Usual Dosage: The usual adult dosage is 500mg-1gm orally before bedtime.
Side Effects: The most common side effect is day time drowsiness.

ETHYL LOFLAZEPATE-CIV (Meilax and Victan)
Prescribed For: The treatment of anxiety.
Drug Class: Benzodiazepines
Usual Dosage: The usual adult dosage is 1mg-3mg orally a day.
Side Effects: The most common side effects are drowsiness, sedation, muscle weakness and

ataxia; less frequently vertigo, headache, confusion, depression, slurred speech, changes in libido, tremor, and visual disturbances.

FENCAMFAMIN-CIV (Reactivan)
Prescribed For: The treatment of depressive fatigue and lethargy.
Drug Class: CNS Drugs & Agents for ADHD
Usual Dosage: The usual adult dosage is 10mg-20mg orally with breakfast and 10mg with lunch if needed.
Side Effects: The most common side effects are dry mouth, restlessness, tremors, and loss of appetite.

FENFLURAMINE HYDROCHLORIDE -CIV (Pondimin)
Prescribed For: The management of exogenous obesity.
Drug Class: Weight loss-supplement
Usual Dosage: The usual adult dosage is the usual dose is one 20 mg tablet three times daily before meals.

Side Effects: The most common side effects are drowsiness, diarrhea, and dry mouth.

FLUDIAZEPAM-CIV (Erispan)
Prescribed For: The treatment of anxiety.
Drug Class: Benzodiazepine Derivative
Usual Dosage: The usual adult dosage is 0.75mg orally a day given in three divided doses.
Side Effects: The most common side effects are respiratory depression, acute pulmonary insufficiency or sleep apnea, and severe hepatic impairment.

FLUNITRAZEPAM-CIV (Rohypnol Tab)
Prescribed For: Pre-medication before surgery and for general anesth.
Drug Class: Benzodiazepine Derivative
Usual Dosage: The usual adult dosage is 0.5mg-1mg orally once a day, with the maximum daily dose being 2mg.

Side Effects: The most common side effects are acute pulmonary insufficiency or sleep apnea, severe hepatic impairment, chronic psychosis, phobic or obsess ional states, may precipitate suicide or aggressive behavior.

FLURAZEPAM-CIV (DALMANE®)
Prescribed For: The treatment of insomnia with characteristic in trouble falling asleep and frequent nocturnal awakenings.
Drug Class: Benzodiazepine Hypnotic Agent
Usual Dosage: The usual adult dosage is 30mg orally at bedtime.
Side Effects: The most common side effects are dizziness, drowsiness, light-headedness, staggering, ataxia and falling.

HALAZEPAM-CIV (Paxipam)
Prescribed For: The short-term treatment of anxiety symptoms.
Drug Class: Benzodiazepines
Usual Dosage: The usual adult starting dosage is 20mg orally three times a day, with maximum daily dose of 160mg.

Side Effects: The most common side effects are dizziness, drowsiness, depression, nausea, vomiting, decreased sex drive, clumsiness, and change in behavior.

KETAZOLAM-CIV (Ansieten, Ansietil, Marcen, Sedatival)
Prescribed For: The short-term treatment of anxiety symptoms.
Drug Class: Benzodiazepines
Usual Dosage: The usual adult dosage is 15mg-30mg orally once a day in the evening.
Side Effects: The most common side effects are CNS depression, fatigue, drowsiness, euphoria, respiratory depression, and dizziness.

LORAZEPAM-CIV (Ativan®)
Prescribed For: The management of anxiety or for the short-term relief from anxiety symptoms.
Drug Class: Anxiolytics, Anticonvulsants, Antivertigo Drugs, and Benzodiazepines
Usual Dosage: The usual adult dosage is 2mg-6mg orally given in

divided doses, with the largest dose given before bedtime.

Side Effects: The most common side effects are CNS depression, fatigue, drowsiness, euphoria, respiratory depression, and dizziness.

LORMETAZEPAM-CIV (Noctamid, Ergocalm, Loramet, Dilamet, Sedaben, Stilaze, Nocton, Pronoctan,)
Prescribed For: It has anxiolytic, anticonvulsant, sedative and skeletal muscle relaxant properties.
Drug Class: Benzodiazepine Derivative
Usual Dosage: The usual adult dosage is 0.5mg-1.5mg orally at bedtime.
Side Effects: The most common side effects are CNS depression, respiratory depression, acute pulmonary insufficiency or sleep apnea, severe hepatic impairment, chronic psychosis, phobic or obsessional states.

MAZINDOL-CIV (Qualizindol Tab)

Prescribed For: The short-term treatment of obesity.
Drug Class: Anti- Obesity Agent
Usual Dosage: The usual adult dosage is 0.5mg-1mg orally every morning for 4-6 weeks.
Side Effects: The most common side effects are severe renal or hepatic impairment cerebrovascular or CV disease, pulmonary artery hypertension, severe arterial hypertension, anorexia nervosa, depression, hyperexcitability and agitation.

MEBUTAMATE-CIV (Capla®)
Prescribed For: Sedative and anxiolytic drug with anti-hypertensive effects.
Drug Class: Barbiturates
Usual Dosage: The usual adult dosage is 300mg orally three times a day.
Side Effects: The most common side effects are dizziness and headaches.

MEDAZEPAM-CIV (Nobrium, Rudotel, Raporan, Ansilan)
Prescribed For: The management of anxiety.

Drug Class: Benzodiazepine Derivative
Usual Dosage: The usual adult dosage is 10mg-30mg orally a day in divided doses.
Side Effects: The most common side effects are fatigue, drowsiness, dizziness, prolonged reaction time, headache, coordination disorders (ataxia), confusion, and anterograde amnesia.

MEPROBAMATE-CIV
Prescribed For: The management of anxiety or for short-term relief of side effects of anxiety.
Drug Class: Carbamate Derivative
Usual Dosage: The usual adult daily dosage is1200 mg to 1600 mg orally in three or four divided doses.
Side Effects: The most common side effects are Drowsiness, ataxia, dizziness, slurred speech, headache, vertigo, weakness, paresthesias, nausea, vomiting, and diarrhea.

METHOHEXITAL-CIV (BREVITAL®)

Prescribed For: The induction of anesthesia prior to the use of other general anesthetic agents.

Drug Class: Barbiturate Anesthetic

Usual Dosage: The usual dosage varies due to weight, height and patients physical condition. Dosage should be given by physician.

Side Effects: The most common side effects are salivation, headache, rhinitis, nausea, emesis, abdominal pain, and respiratory depression.

MEPHOBARBITAL-CIV (MEBARAL)

Prescribed For: The treatment of anxiety, tension, apprehension, and preventing seizures.

Drug Class: Barbiturate

Usual Dosage: The usual adult dosage is 400mg-600mg orally daily. For children under the age of 5 years old is 16mg-32mg orally three to four times daily.

Side Effects: The most common side effects are agitation, confusion, hyperkinesia, ataxia, CNS depression, nightmares, nervousness, psychiatric disturbance, hallucinations, insomnia, anxiety, dizziness, thinking abnormality.

MIDAZOLAM INJECTION-CIV (VERSED)
Prescribed For: The sedation before therapeutic or endoscopic procedures, and also as a general anesthesia.
Drug Class: Benzodiazepine
Usual Dosage: The usual dosage varies due to weight, height and patients physical condition. Dosage should be given by physician.
Side Effects: The most common side effects are nausea, vomiting, coughing, headache, and drowsiness.

MODAFINIL-CIV (Provigil)
Prescribed For: The treatment of wakefulness in patients that suffer from sleepiness linked to narcolepsy.
Drug Class: Wakefulness-Promoting Agent
Usual Dosage: The usual adult dosage is 200mg orally once a day.
Side Effects: The most common side effects are headache, nausea,

nervousness, rhinitis, diarrhea, back pain, anxiety, insomnia, dizziness, and dyspepsia.

NIMETAZEPAM-IV (Erimin)
Prescribed For: The treatment of insomnia, and also as a muscle relaxant.
Drug Class: Benzodiazepine Derivative
Usual Dosage: The usual adult dosage is 5mg tablet orally.
Side Effects: The most common side effects are drowsiness, dizziness, lightheadedness, fatigue, or loss of coordination.

NITRAZEPAM-CIV (Alodorm, Arem, Insoma, and Mogadon)
Prescribed For: Hypnotic and sedative use.
Drug Class: Benzodiazepine
Usual Dosage: The usual adult dosage ranges between 5mg-10mg tablets orally.
Side Effects: The most common side effects are drowsiness, dizziness, lightheadedness, fatigue, or loss of coordination.

OXAZEPAM-CIV (Serax®)
Prescribed For: The management of anxiety or short-term relief of symptoms of anxiety.
Drug Class: Benzodiazepines
Usual Dosage: The usual adult dosage for mild to moderate anxiety it is 10mg-15mg orally 3-4 times a day. For severe anxiety it is 15mg-30mg orally 3-4 times a day.
Side Effects: The most common side effects are dizziness, vertigo, headache, and nausea.

PARALDEHYDE-CIV (PARAL)
Prescribed For: The treatment of certain convulsive disorders.
Drug Class: Anticonvulsant
Usual Dosage: The usual adult's dosage varies in patients according to body weight, height, and physical condition. Dosage should be determined by physicians.
Side Effects: The most common side effects are coughing, rash, yellowing of the eyes or skin, and redness or swelling at the injection site.

PEMOLINE-CIV (Cylert)
Prescribed For: The treatment of
Attention Deficit Hyperactivity
Disorder (ADHD).
**Drug Class: Central Nervous
System Stimulant**
Usual Dosage: The usual starting
dosage is one 37.5mg tablet orally
once a day in the morning. Then
may be increased by 18.75mg one
week at a time.
Side Effects: The most common
side effects are hallucinations,
dyskinetic movements of the
tongue, lips, face and extremities,
abnormal oculomotor function
including nystagmus and oculogyric
crisis, mild depression, dizziness,
increased irritability, headache,
drowsiness, and insomnia.

**PENTAZOCINE-CIV
(TALWIN®)**
Prescribed For: For the relief of
moderate to severe pain.
Drug Class: Benzazocine
Usual Dosage: The usual adult
dosage is one tablet every three to
four hours.
Side Effects: The most common
side effects are hypertension,

hypotension, circulatory depression, tachycardia, syncope, and respiratory.

PHENOBARBITAL-CIV
Prescribed For: The short-term treatment of insomnia, sedatives, and long-term anticonvulsants for the treatment of generalized tonic-clonic and cortical local seizures.
Drug Class: Barbiturate, Nonselective Central Nervous System Depressant
Usual Dosage: The usual adult dosage for daytime sedative is 30mg-120mg orally daily in 2-3 divided doses. For a bedtime hypnotic 100mg to 320mg orally. Also for use as an anticonvulsant is 50mg -100mg orally 2-3 times daily.
Side Effects: The most common side effects are agitation, confusion, hyperkinesia, ataxia, CNS depression, nightmares, nervousness, psychiatric disturbance, hallucinations, insomnia, anxiety, dizziness, thinking abnormality.

PHENTERMINE-CIV (Adipex-P®)

Prescribed For: Short-term use in a weight loss regimen with exercise, and a healthily balanced diet.

Drug Class: Weight control supplement

Usual Dosage: The usual dosage is 37.5mg orally before breakfast or 1-2 hours after breakfast. The dosage maybe reduced for some patients.

Side Effects: The most common side effects are palpitation, tachycardia, elevation of blood pressure, over stimulation, restlessness, dizziness, insomnia, euphoria, dysphoria, tremor, and headache.

PINAZEPAM-CIV (DOMAR CAP)

Prescribed For: The treatment of anxiety and insomnia.

Drug Class: Benzodiazepine Derivative

Usual Dosage: The usual dosage for anxiety is 5mg-20mg orally in divided doses. For insomnia 2.5mg-5mg orally at bedtime.

Side Effects: The most common side effects are acute pulmonary insufficiency, myasthenia gravis, sleep apnea, severe hepatic impairment, drowsiness, sedation, muscle weakness and ataxia less frequently vertigo, headache, confusion, depression, slurred speech, changes in libido, and tremors.

PIPRADROL-CIV (MERETRAN)
Prescribed For: The treatment of narcolepsy, ADHD, and senile dementia.
Drug Class: Mild Central Nervous System Stimulant
Usual Dosage: The usual dosage is between 0.5mg -4mg orally once a day in the morning.
Side Effects: The most common side effects include insomnia, anorexia, tachycardia, anxiety.

PRAZEPAM-CIV (CENTRAX)
Prescribed For: The treatment of anxiety.
Drug Class: Benzodiazepine Derivative Drug

Usual Dosage: The usual dose is 15mg-30mg orally at bedtime. For severe cases 60mg maybe taken.

Side Effects: The most common side effects are respiratory depression, acute pulmonary insufficiency or sleep apnea, severe hepatic impairment, chronic psychosis, phobic or obsessional state, glaucoma, and porphyria.

PROPOXYPHENE HYDROCHLORIDE–CIV (Darvon)

Prescribed For: Mild to moderate pain relief.

Drug Class: Opioid Analgesic

Usual Dosage: The usual adult dosage is 65mg orally every four hours as needed for pain.

Side Effects: The most common side effects are constipation, lightheadedness, dizziness, drowsiness, stomach upset, nausea, and flushing or vision changes.

PROPOXYPHENE NAPSYLATE WITH ACETAMINOPHEN-CIV (Darvocet-N)

Prescribed For: For the relief of mild to moderate pain, either when pain is present alone or when it is accompanied by fever.
Drug Class: Opioid Analgesic
Usual Dosage: The usual adult dosage is 100 mg propoxyphene napsylate and 650 mg acetaminophen orally every 4 hours as needed for pain.
Side Effects: The most common side effects are constipation, lightheadedness, headache, dizziness, sedation, nausea, and vomiting.

QUAZEPAM-CIV (DORAL)
Prescribed For: Treatment of insomnia caused by difficulty falling asleep, and frequently wakening during sleeping.
Drug Class: Benzodiazepine Hypnotic Agent
Usual Dosage: The starting dose is 15mg orally at bedtime, but may be reduced to 7.5mg for some patients.
Side Effects: The most common side effects are drowsiness, headache, depression, nervousness, agitation, amnesia, anorexia,

anxiety, apathy, euphoria, impotence, decreased libido, paranoid reaction, nightmares, and abnormal thinking.

SIBUTRAMINE HYDROCHLORIDE MONOHYDRATE-CIV (MERIDIA)
Prescribed For: The management of obesity including weight loss.
Drug Class: Weight Loss Agent
Usual Dosage: The starting dose is 10mg orally once a day and may be titrated there after.
Side Effects: The most common side effects are dry mouth, anorexia, insomnia, constipation and headache.

TEMAZEPAM-CIV (Restoril™)
Prescribed For: The short-term treatment of insomnia.
Drug Class: Benzodiazepine Hypnotic Agent
Usual Dosage: The recommended adult's dose is 15mg orally at bedtime.
Side Effects: The most common side effects are drowsiness,

headache, fatigue, depression, dry mouth, and euphoria.

TETRAZEPAM-CIV (Clinoxan, Epsipam, Myolastan, Musaril, Relaxam and Spasmorela)
Prescribed For: The treatment of muscle spasm, anxiety disorders such as panic attacks, or more rarely to treat depression, premenstrual syndrome or agoraphobia.
Drug Class: Benzodiazepine Derivative
Usual Dosage: The recommended adult dose for muscle spasm is 50 mg three to four times per day.
Side Effects: The most common side effects are drowsiness, fatigue, and unsteadiness.

TRIAZOLAM-CIV (Halcion®)
Prescribed For: The short-term treatment of insomnia, usually 7-10 days.
Drug Class: Triazolobenzodiazepine Hypnotic Agent
Usual Dosage: The recommended dose for most adults is 0.25 mg orally at bedtime. For patients with

low body weight may take a dose of 0.125mg. The maximum daily dose is 0.5mg.

Side Effects: The most common side effects are drowsiness, dizziness, or light-headedness.

ZALEPLON-CIV (Sonata®)

Prescribed For: The short-term treatment of insomnia.

Drug Class: Nonbenzodiazepine Hypnotic

Usual Dosage: The recommended dose for adults is 10mg orally at bedtime. Doses should not exceed 20mg/day.

Side Effects: The most common side effects are back pain, chest pain, fever, and chest pain substernal, chills, face edema, generalized edema, hangover effect, neck rigidity, migraine, constipation, dry mouth, and dyspepsia.

ZOLPIDEM-CIV (Ambien, Zolpimist)

Prescribed For: The treatment of insomnia.

Drug Class: Sedatives or Hypnotics

Usual Dosage: The recommended dose for adults is 10 mg orally once daily immediately before bedtime. The total dose should not exceed 10 mg per day.

Side Effects: The most common side effects are drowsiness, dizziness, euphoria, confusion, insomnia, euphoria, ataxia (balance problems), and visual changes.

ZOPICLONE-CIV (Imovane, Zimovane and Zopinox)

Prescribed For: The treatment of insomnia.

Drug Class: Cyclopyrrolone Derivative

Usual Dosage: The usual dosage is 5mg-20 mg and 7.5 mg, respectively.

Side Effects: Include daytime drowsiness, dizziness, lightheadedness, bitter taste, dry mouth, headache or stomach upset may occur the first few days as your body adjusts to the medication.

GUAIFENSIN AND CODEINE-CV (Robitussin Ac)

Prescribed For: The temporary control of coughs due to minor throat and bronchial irritation as may occur with the common cold or inhaled irritants, and also helps remove mucus.

Drug Class: Cough Suppressant

Usual Dosage: The usual adult dosage is 2 teaspoonfuls orally every 4 hours, not to exceed 12 teaspoonfuls in a 24-hour period.

Side Effects: The most common side effects are dizziness, drowsiness, excitability, headache, nausea, nervousness or anxiety, trouble sleeping and weakness.

PREGABALIN-CV (LYRICA)

Prescribed For: The control of neuropathic pain associated with diabetic peripheral neuropathy, and fibromyalgia.

Drug Class: Antiepileptic

Usual Dosage: The usual dosage for postherpetic neuralgia is 75 mg twice daily or 50 mg three times daily. The dose may be increased to 100 mg 3 times daily (300 mg/day) after one week. For fibromyalgia 300-450 mg/day in 2 or 3 divided doses.

Side Effects: The most common side effects of pregabalin are dizziness, drowsiness, dry mouth, edema (accumulation of fluid), blurred vision, weight gain, and difficulty concentrating. Other side effects include reduced blood platelet counts, and increased blood creatinine kinase levels.

PROMETHAZINE WITH CODEINE-CV (Phenergan with Codeine)
Prescribed For: The temporary relief of cough and upper respiratory symptoms associated with allergy or the common cold.
Drug Class: Cough Suppressant
Usual Dosage: The usual adult dosage is 5ml orally every 4-6 hours, not exceeding 30ml in 24 hours.
Side Effects: The most common side effects are stomach upset, nausea, vomiting, constipation, dizziness, drowsiness or headache.

200 Top Prescribed Medications in the United States as of 2009

1. Hydrocodone with acetaminophen
2. Lipitor
3. Atenolol
4. Synthroid
5. Premarin
6. Zithromax
7. Furosemide
8. Amoxicillin
9. Norvasc
10. Hydrochlorothiazide
11. Alprazolam
12. Albuterol
13. Zoloft
14. Paxil
15. Zocor
16. Prevacid
17. Ibuprofen
18. Triamterene with Hydrochlorothiazide
19. Toprol-XL
20. Cephalexin
21. Celebrex
22. Zyrtec
23. Levoxyl
24. Allegra
25. Ortho Tri-Cyclen
26. Celexa
27. Prednisone
28. Prilosec
29. Claritin
30. Fluoxetine
31. Acetaminophen with codeine
32. Ambien
33. Metoprolol

34. Lorazepam
35. Fosamax
36. Propoxyphene-N with acetaminophen
37. Metformin
38. Ranitidine
39. Amitriptyline
40. Viagra
41. Prempro
42. Trimox
43. Neurontin
44. Wellbutrin SR
45. Pravachol
46. Augmentin
47. Nexium
48. Accupril
49. Lisinopril
50. Effexor XR
51. Singulair
52. Zestril
53. Potassium chloride
54. Clonazepam
55. Naproxen
56. Warfarin
57. Trazodone
58. Cipro
59. Flonase
60. Cyclobenzaprine
61. Verapamil
62. Enalapril
63. Albuterol
64. Isosorbide mononitrate
65. Levaquin
66. Diazepam
67. Glucotrol XL
68. Coumadin
69. Plavix
70. Diflucan

71. Advair Diskus
72. Protonix
73. Lotrel
74. Amoxil
75. Diovan
76. Glyburide
77. Carisoprodol
78. Altace
79. Allopurinol
80. Estradiol
81. Avandia
82. Actos
83. Lotensin
84. Clarinex
85. Medroxyprogesterone
86. Oxycodone with acetaminophen
87. Doxycycline
88. Lanoxin
89. Cozaar
90. Nasonex
91. Diltiazem
92. Clonidine
93. Prinivil
94. Digitek
95. Methylprednisolone
96. Evista
97. Folic acid
98. Glucophage XR
99. Penicillin VK
100. Flovent
101. Risperdal
102. Cotrim
103. Promethazine with codeine
104. Diovan HCT
105. Aciphex
106. Zyprexa
107. Allegra-D

108. Levothroid
109. Doxazosin
110. Xalatan
111. Gemfibrozil
112. Flomax
113. Temazepam
114. Ultram
115. Hyzaar
116. OxyContin
117. Humulin N
118. Depakote
119. Concerta
120. Klor-Con
121. Glucovance
122. Imitrex
123. Terazosin
124. Claritin D 24HR
125. Cartia XT
126. Amaryl
127. Spironolactone
128. TriCor
129. Ortho-Novum
130. Hydroxyzine
131. Monopril
132. Combivent
133. Meclizine
134. Triamcinolone
135. Klor-Con M20
136. Metoclopramide
137. Minocycline
138. Bisoprolol with Hydrochlorothiazide
139. Propranolol
140. Glucophage
141. Propacet
142. Valtrex
143. Remeron
144. Famotidine

145. Metronidazole
146. Avapro
147. Glipizide
148. Buspirone
149. Nystatin
150. Skelaxin
151. Serevent
152. Dilantin
153. Promethazine/Codeine
154. Necon
155. Captopril
156. Clindamycin
157. Aspirin
158. Seroquel
159. Acyclovir
160. Macrobid
161. Claritin D 12HR
162. Amoxicillin with potassium clavulanate
163. Adderall XR
164. Biaxin XL
165. Trivora-28
166. Ortho-Cyclen
167. Cefzil
168. Humulin 70/30
169. Detrol LA
170. Coreg
171. Tiazac
172. Biaxin
173. Tramadol
174. Nasacort AQ
175. Humalog
176. Ultracet
177. Endocet
178. Bactroban
179. Veetids
180. Sulfamethoxazole with trimethoprim
181. Timolol

182. Rhinocort Aqua
183. Claritin Reditabs
184. Nortriptyline
185. Aviane

186. Actonel
187. Topamax
188. Microgestin Fe
189. Tamoxifen
190. Mircette
191. Nifedipine
192. Ditropan XL
193. Tetracycline
194. Apri
195. Zestoretic
196. Diclofenac
197. Augmentin ES
198. Carbidopa with levodopa
199. Nabumetone
200. Hydrocritsone

Medical Abbreviations

aa	of each
a.c.	before meals
a.d.	right ear
ad	as desired
a.l.	left ear
AM	morning
Amt	amount
aq.	water. aqueous
a.u.	each ear
b.i.d.	twice a day
B.P.	blood pressure
cap	capsule
cath	catheter
C.B.C	complete blood count
cc.	cubic centimeter
chol	cholesterol
cm	centimeter
c/o	complains of
comp	compounded of
CV	cardiovascular
dil	dilute
disch	discharge
disp	dispensary
dr	dram
Dx	diagnosis
etc.	and so on
exp	expired
ext	extract, external
fl. dr.	fluidram

fl. oz. fluid ounce
ft.   let there be made
gm.   gram
gr.   grain
gtt.   a drop or drops
hr.   hour
h.s.   at bedtime
hypo hypodermic syringe or injection
H2O water
inj   injection
I.V. intravenous
k   kilogram
L   liter, left, put left first
lb.   pound
mcg. microgram
mEq. milliequivalent
mg.   milliliter
mm.   millimeter
No.   number
Noct. night
NR   no refill
o.d. right eye
o.s. left eye
o.u. each eye
oz.   ounce
p   pulse, pint
p.c. after meals
PM   afternoon, evening
P.O. by mouth
p.r.n as needed
pt   patient, pint

pulv. powder
q4h   every 4 hours
q.d.   every day
q.h.   every hour
qid   four times a day
qod   every other day
qt.   quart
Rx   a prescription
sol.   solution
solv. dissolve
sos   if necessary or required
stat   immediately
syr.   syrup
tab   tablet
tbsp. tablespoonful
tid   three times a day
TPN total parenteral nutrition
tsp.   teaspoonful
ung. ointment
vol.   volume
wt   weight

Conversion Factors

To convert:

Milligrams per kilogram to milligrams per pound, multiply by .45
Milligrams per kilogram to grains per pound, multiply by .007
Milligrams per pound to grains per pound, multiply by .015
Grains per pound to milligrams per pound, multiply by 65
Grains per pound to milligrams per kilogram, multiply by 143
Fahrenheit degrees into Celsius, subtract 32, multiply by 5 and divide by 9
Celsius degrees into Fahrenheit, multiply by 9, divide by 5 and add 32

Conversions for Weights, Measures and Equivalents
(These are approximate conversions)

1 kilogram	**= 1,000 grams**
1 gram	**= 1,000 milligrams**
1 milligram	**= 1,000 micrograms**
60 milligrams	**= 1 grain**
28.35 grams	**= 1 ounce**

1 kilogram	= 2.2 pounds
454 grams	= 1 pound
1 millimeter	= 0.04 inches
1 centimeter	= .4 inches
2.5 centimeter	= 1 inch
1 meter	= 39.37 inches
1 liter	= 1,000 cubic centimeters
1 liter	= 1.000 milliliters
30 milliliters	= 1 fluid ounce
20 drops	= 1 milliliter
1 teaspoon	= 5 milliliters
1 tablespoon	= 15 milliliters
16 ounces	= 1 pint
2 pints	= 1 quart
4 quarts	= 1 gallon
1 pint	= 473 milliliters

INDEX

INDEX

INDEX

INDEX

INDEX

81

INDEX

* 9 7 8 0 9 8 2 0 2 1 5 1 4 *